LIVING WITH DISEASE

PARKINSON'S DISEASE

BY LORI DITTMER

CREATIVE EDUCATION

Contents

CHAPTERS

Introduction 4

1 THE "SHAKING PALSY" 6

2 THE DOPAMINE CONNECTION 16

3 LIFE WITH PARKINSON'S 26

4 COMMITTED TO A CURE 36

SIDEBARS

Parkinson's Strikes the Greatest 12

Acting the Part 22

Discovering Levodopa 28

All in the Family 42

Glossary 46

Bibliography 47

Further Reading 47

Index 48

When Brian Grant, a retired

National Basketball Association (NBA) player, first noticed a tremor in his left hand, a **neurologist** told him it was the result of stress. Grant eagerly accepted the diagnosis; after all, the 6-foot-9 and 254-pound athlete had made his living off his muscle coordination and control. He did not want to believe that anything more serious might be wrong. When the tremor did not go away, Grant tried to hide it. For example, while coaching his sons' basketball teams, he dribbled to occupy his hand. But after months of trying to disguise it, he sought a second opinion and was diagnosed with young-onset Parkinson's disease. In May 2009, at the age of 37, Grant made public his condition and joined the fight to raise awareness of the disease. Although researchers do not know what causes some people to develop Parkinson's, much has been discovered about how the disease affects the brain, enabling scientists to produce therapies that ease the symptoms from which patients suffer.

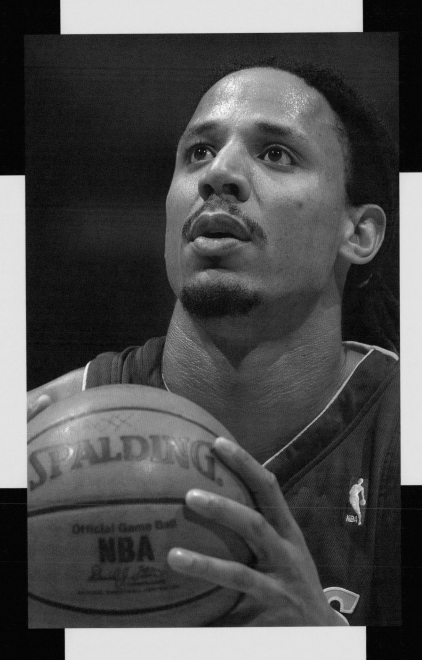

In 2004–05, Brian Grant's last full NBA season, he played for the Los Angeles Lakers.

CHAPTER ONE

THE "SHAKING PALSY"

In the early 1800s, a London doctor

named James Parkinson began writing about a disease he observed in several of his patients and other people in his neighborhood. Each displayed varying degrees of **involuntary** trembling in a hand or an arm, and some stooped forward, taking short, quick steps as they walked. Parkinson called the disease the "shaking palsy," and in 1817, he published a medical paper based on what he had learned about it. Although physicians had noted the shaking palsy for centuries, Parkinson was one of the first to study it. Sixty years later, Jean Martin Charot, a French neurologist, continued Parkinson's work, honoring the doctor's foresight by changing the name of the ailment to Parkinson's disease.

After Parkinson's groundbreaking essay, research on the disease crept along slowly. Until the medication levodopa became available in the 1960s, the **prognosis** for a patient with Parkinson's disease was grim. The disease eventually made movement impossible, leaving patients unable to eat, fight off other diseases or infections, or even get out of bed.

In addition to practicing medicine, James Parkinson also lectured on political and social matters of the day.

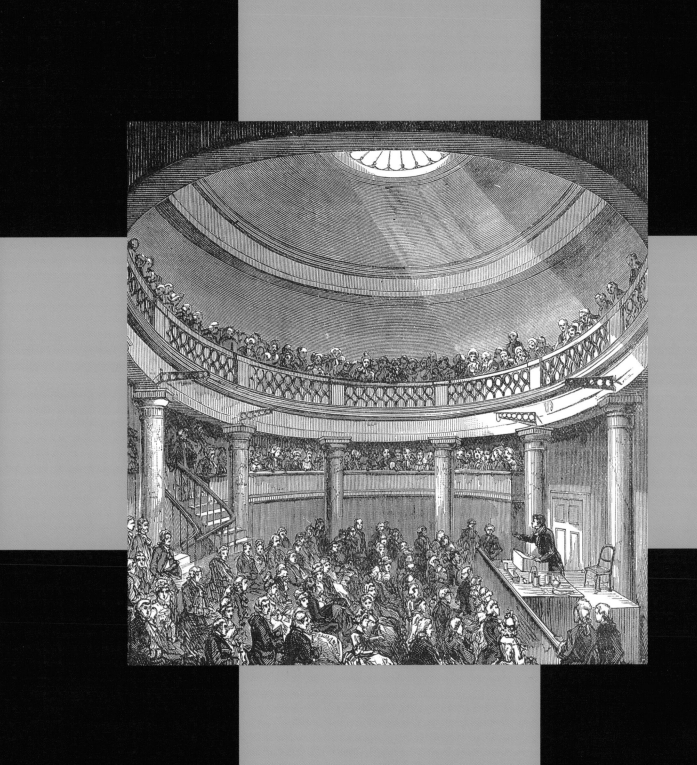

Since Parkinson's time, most researchers have considered the disease that bears his name to be a movement disorder. The brain loses control over how and when the body's muscles work. As a result, people with Parkinson's struggle with involuntary movements and often feel stiff or "frozen." But Parkinson's patients face challenges that go deeper than physical movement. Some also develop memory and thinking problems, as well as depression, which can lead to loneliness and social isolation.

Today, about 1 million people in North America have Parkinson's disease, and about 60,000 more cases are diagnosed each year. Worldwide, more than 4 million people suffer from the disease. People can develop Parkinson's at any age, but on average, patients learn they have the disease around age 60. Young-onset Parkinson's disease occurs in people younger than 40. Only about 5 to 10 percent of all people with Parkinson's have this form of the disease. Parkinson's disease is not infectious, but scientists have yet to discover its cause. The disease is **chronic** and **degenerative**, which means that it will never go away and that its symptoms will continue to worsen throughout the patient's life.

For about 70 percent of people with Parkinson's, the first noticeable symptom—the one that prompts them to visit the doctor—is a tremor, or an uncontrollable, rhythmic shaking in a finger, hand, or foot

Forty to 50 percent of Parkinson's patients report suffering from depression, and another 25 to 40 percent experience anxiety or nervousness. About half of Parkinson's patients deal with fatigue, and 40 percent show apathy, or a loss of interest and enthusiasm for the things that once brought them joy. About 30 percent of Parkinson's patients eventually develop dementia.

on just one side of the body. The Parkinson's tremor is also referred to as a resting tremor, since it is more obvious when a person is not trying to move the body part. Once the person begins to use the affected hand or foot, the tremor subsides.

Because doctors have no test to reveal that a patient is suffering from Parkinson's disease, scientists cannot conclusively confirm a diagnosis until after the patient dies. Then researchers can examine the patient's brain to look for the physical damage caused by the disease. In the absence of a test, most physicians who suspect a case of Parkinson's will wait to see how the symptoms change or progress. At the same time, the doctor will perform a variety of tests to rule out other conditions, such as a brain tumor or multiple sclerosis (a disease that causes increasing muscle weakness and loss of coordination).

To come to a diagnosis of Parkinson's disease, doctors generally look for four signs. Having two of these four signs may indicate the presence of Parkinson's; tremor, rigidity, slowness of movement, and a loss of balance. Only about 15 percent of Parkinson's patients do not have the hallmark symptom of a tremor. However, young-onset patients may experience slowness of movement and a tingling sensation in the hands and feet as initial symptoms instead.

PARKINSON'S DISEASE

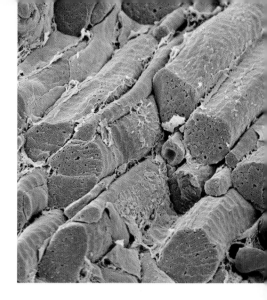

Rigidity is a condition that occurs when muscles can no longer move **spontaneously** or relax normally. This noticeably affects facial muscles, often leaving Parkinson's patients with a masked face that is unable to smile or show emotion as easily as it did in the past. Patients can display two types of rigidity. In someone with lead-pipe rigidity, the muscles become so tense and resistant to movement that bending them takes enormous effort—almost like trying to bend a lead pipe. A person with cogwheel rigidity can no longer bend an arm or leg smoothly but instead uses jerky motions. Rigid muscles also cause what is known as frozen shoulder, a painful stiffness in the shoulder commonly reported by people with Parkinson's.

Slowness of movement can also be a sign of Parkinson's disease. Previously effortless motions, such as brushing teeth, tying shoes, or even blinking, become difficult. Some people have problems getting their feet to take a step or have difficulty saying a word. Even the movement of the digestive system slows down, which can lead to choking, stomachache, and constipation, as the sluggish intestinal muscles do not efficiently move waste out of the body. Performing two tasks at the same time becomes nearly impossible. As the disease progresses, some

Skeletal muscle has a uniquely cylindrical shape and is attached at two points to the skeleton.

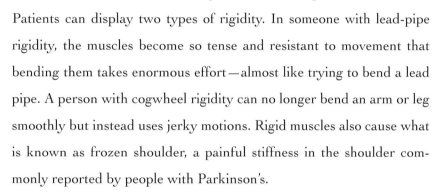

Parkinson's Strikes the Greatest

Born in 1942 as Cassius Clay, boxer Muhammad Ali began fighting when he was just 12 years old. He went on to win the light-heavyweight gold medal at the 1960 Olympic Games. Never shy about self-promotion, Ali called himself "The Greatest" and recited rhymes to predict the round in which he would beat his opponent. Ali retired in 1981 with a lifetime record of 56–5. By then, the years of receiving blows to the head had taken a toll on his body. He announced his struggle with Parkinson's in 1984. Gradually, Ali's voice softened to a whisper, his movement and speech slowed, and tremors overtook his body. With a sharp mind but a frail body, Ali made a rare public appearance in December 2009 at the opening of the Muhammad Ali Parkinson Center in Phoenix, Arizona. The center was described as the country's most comprehensive facility for treating Parkinson's disease to date.

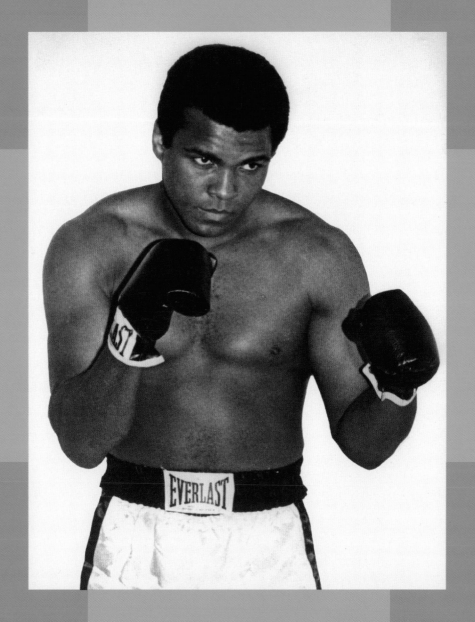

In 1960, Muhammad Ali was on the cusp of greatness, winning two other amateur titles besides the Olympic medal.

movements may stop altogether. For example, one arm might not swing while the person walks. Muscle slowness can also cause changes in the handwriting of a Parkinson's patient. Although the first few letters might flow normally, the person's hand begins to cramp and tighten, resulting in shrinking penmanship. Due to the changes in Adolf Hitler's handwriting over time, historians have **hypothesized** that the German dictator had Parkinson's disease.

The fourth sign of Parkinson's is a loss of balance. As their balance gets worse, many Parkinson's patients stoop or lean forward as they walk, which can lead to stumbling or falling. Patients may take short, shuffling steps and grasp at doorknobs and handrails to maintain their balance.

In addition, many Parkinson's patients report that they have lost most or all of their sense of smell. Some suffer from excessive sweating, a skin rash on the scalp and face, or nighttime drooling that soaks their pillow.

Not everyone with signs of Parkinson's has the disease, though. Symptoms such as slow movements and balance problems can be the result of a **stroke** or a side effect of medication. Features of Parkinson's that may be applied to other disorders are called "parkinsonism."

After Alzheimer's disease, Parkinson's is the most common progressive disease of the nervous system in the U.S. Researchers estimate that up to 5.3 million Americans have Alzheimer's, while about 1 million suffer from Parkinson's. An estimated 400,000 have multiple sclerosis, another disease of the nervous system.

CHAPTER TWO

THE DOPAMINE CONNECTION

The space between two nerve cells across which neurotransmitters send messages is called a synapse.

Parkinson's disease develops within the brain years before its victim ever realizes what is happening. Deep inside the brain, just above the spinal cord, sit two cell masses called the substantia nigra (Latin for "black substance"). There is one substantia nigra on each side of the brain, and these areas are important for control of body movement.

Cells in the substantia nigra produce dopamine, which is a neurotransmitter, or a chemical that sends signals between nerve cells. The nerve cells, in turn, carry messages to different parts of the brain. Nerve cells use dopamine to communicate with one another and to tell other parts of the body what to do. There are many activities humans perform without so much as thinking about them. We can walk, talk, and blink without concentrating specifically on carrying out those tasks. Dopamine keeps these **unconscious** systems in check by communicating between the brain and muscles.

In people with Parkinson's, the dopamine-producing nerve cells die. As the cells degenerate, the substantia nigra lose their black pigment,

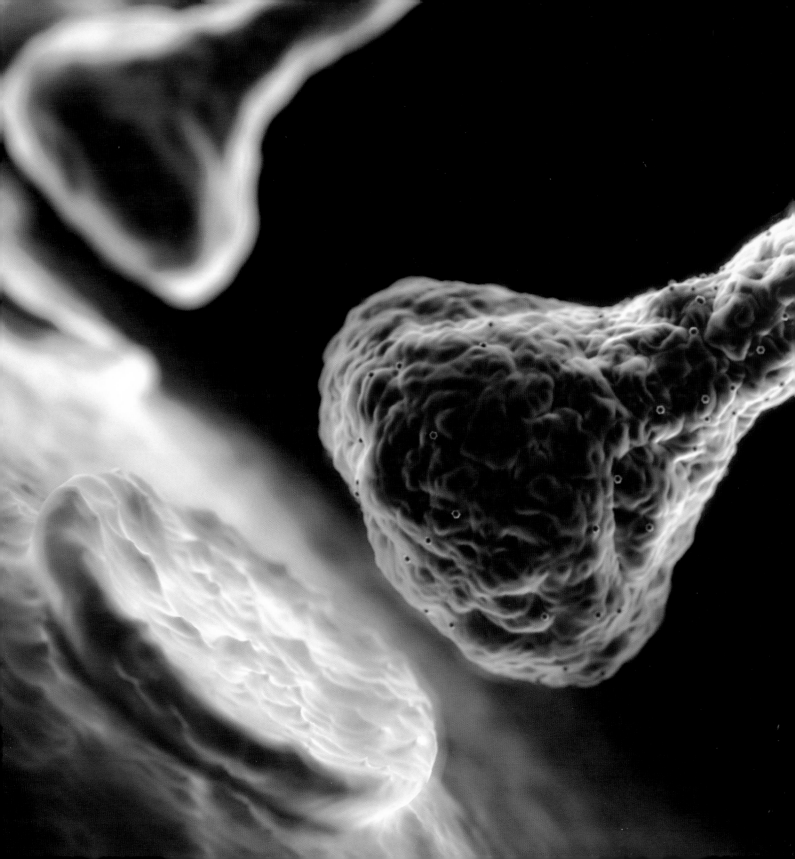

or coloring. They also gradually lose the ability to make dopamine, and communication between the brain and muscles breaks down. When the majority of the dopamine-producing cells in the substantia nigra have died, the muscles begin acting strangely—tightening, moving more slowly, or failing to move at all. The less dopamine available, the more severe the problems become.

By the time a person starts to notice the symptoms of Parkinson's disease, up to 80 percent of the nerve cells have died. Researchers have focused their attention on the lack of dopamine in Parkinson's patients because that is the shortage that produces the most notable change in the brain. However, other neurotransmitters can also be affected. Nor-epinephrine, which is involved in controlling blood vessels and the heart, and serotonin, which helps control sleep, memory, and mood, also break down and become depleted in Parkinson's patients.

The protein deposits known as Lewy bodies were named for their discoverer, Friederich H. Lewy.

Another change in the brains of people with Parkinson's disease is the development of Lewy bodies. These are clumps of **protein** within some nerve cells in the brain, but what they do remains a mystery. Some researchers believe that Lewy bodies, which can be seen only with a microscope in an **autopsy**, lead to dementia in Parkinson's patients.

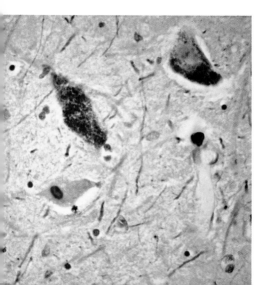

So far, scientists have been unable to determine what triggers the death of dopamine-producing cells. Studies on families of people with Parkinson's have uncovered seven **genes** that play a role in some instances of the disease, particularly in younger people. Researchers think that severe head trauma, such as repeated blows to the head or unconsciousness, may also cause some cases of Parkinson's. In addition, environmental factors may damage the substantia nigra. Pesticides, fertilizers, and metals such as manganese, mercury, and lead have been suspected of triggering Parkinson's by damaging or causing inflammation in the brain's nerve cells. Studies have suggested that Vietnam War and Persian Gulf War veterans who were exposed to high levels of **toxins**, including nerve gas weapons and pesticides, have a higher rate of Parkinson's disease than is otherwise present in the general public. In addition, the rate of Parkinson's disease in the United States appears to be higher in midwestern states, where farming is prevalent. Farmers often use pesticides and other chemicals to protect and nurture their crops.

Because their minds and bodies are still growing and forming, children are particularly vulnerable to the effects of chemicals and toxins, and exposure as a child may affect the brain as an adult. Some researchers believe that if a **fetus** is exposed to toxins, it will never develop fully

Parkinson's disease affects 1 out of every 100 Americans over the age of 60. Most cases of Parkinson's are not inherited, but researchers estimate that 10 to 15 percent of those with the disease have a family member who suffers from it.

functioning substantia nigra. The child might be able to produce enough dopamine for a few decades before a decline begins. Other scientists theorize that a series of toxic exposures throughout a person's life can injure an ever-increasing number of cells until not enough remain to make dopamine.

A more popular explanation for the cause of Parkinson's combines genetics and the environment. Some people might inherit a **predisposition** to Parkinson's, but they might never develop the disease, unless they are exposed to something in the environment that sets it in motion.

Regardless of Parkinson's causes, it is a disease that only gets worse over time. Physicians use rating scales to determine the severity of the symptoms and better understand and treat their Parkinson's patients accordingly. The Unified Parkinson's Disease Rating Scale is a **comprehensive** evaluation that enables doctors to evaluate patients on physical disabilities as well as challenges with non-motor activities, such as speech, memory, and mood. A neurologist asks the patient to perform certain tasks and scores the patient's performance from 0 (normal) to 4 (severe). The higher the number, the greater the disability.

The Hoehn and Yahr scale is a shorter test that divides the progress of Parkinson's into five stages based on the physical changes a Parkin-

Acting the Part

A rising star in Hollywood, Michael J. Fox had appeared in the 1980s television sitcom *Family Ties* and hit movies such as *Back to the Future* before he woke up one morning with a twitching left pinkie finger. When the twitching did not go away, Fox went to the doctor. He was just 30 years old when he was diagnosed with young-onset Parkinson's in 1991, though it is possible that his disease had gone unnoticed for up to 10 years. For several years afterward, Fox hid his disease with the help of medicine and surgery to reduce both the tremors and the stiffness that had overtaken the left side of his body. He finally publicly announced his struggle with Parkinson's in 1998 and began the quest for a cure. With the help of medication to control his tremors, slurred speech, and frozen facial muscles, Fox has continued to appear in guest roles on television and has provided the voice for characters in animated movies.

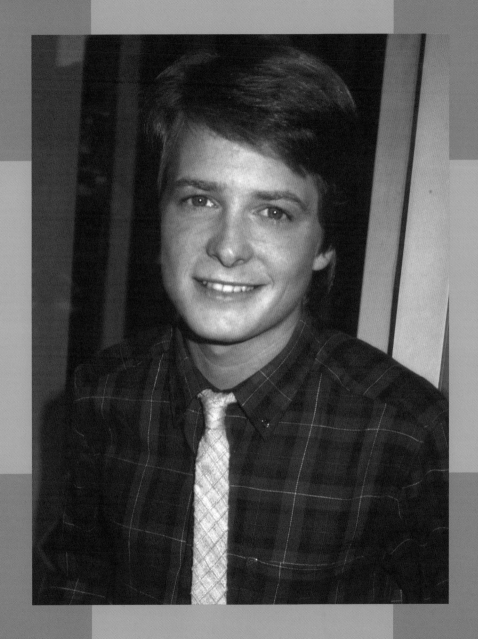

In 1984, Michael J. Fox was two years into his Emmy Award-winning role as Alex Keaton on *Family Ties*.

BY THE NUMBERS **According to the National Vital Statistics Report, complications stemming from Parkinson's disease ranked 14th among the leading causes of death in the U.S. for 2006. Diseases of the heart topped the list, accounting for 631,636 deaths. Parkinson's was blamed for 19,566 deaths.**

son's patient would experience in the absence of treatment or therapy to help control symptoms. The length of time between stages varies from person to person. In Stage One, symptoms—most often a tremor—have begun on one side of the body. Although these symptoms may bother the person with the disease, they don't prevent daily activities. By Stage Two, patients still have minimal disability, but the symptoms have spread to both sides of the body. At Stage Three, Parkinson's causes more serious balance problems and slowness in movement. Although people in Stage Four can stand and walk a little without help, they can no longer live alone because they need assistance with one or more aspects of daily life, such as dressing, bathing, or eating. Rigidity and slowness become much worse, but the tremor might subside. By Stage Five, patients become bedridden or wheelchair-bound and need nursing care.

People do not die from Parkinson's directly, but they can develop serious disabilities and dangerous complications that can lead to death. Many patients have problems swallowing and choke easily on their food. Others have such poor balance that they are prone to falling. A bad fall can cause broken bones that don't heal properly, allowing dangerous infections to set in. Since the disease affects people in different ways, some patients can live for up to 15 years before their symptoms grow severe. With the help of medication, some might never become severely disabled.

CHAPTER THREE

LIFE WITH PARKINSON'S

Because there is no cure for

Parkinson's disease, patients do not recover from it. As symptoms grow worse, people must learn to cope with the condition. Slowly, people with Parkinson's lose their fine motor skills. In other words, tasks that require repetitive motions—such as brushing teeth, working with small objects, buttoning a shirt, or applying makeup—can become nearly impossible.

Occupational therapy can help Parkinson's patients learn new ways to perform daily tasks, such as getting out of bed by rocking back and forth and swinging the arms and legs to one side. Occupational therapists can also recommend devices to help patients move around safely at home. Installing tub and shower grab bars and using aids such as walkers and canes might be humiliating for some people, especially those with young-onset Parkinson's, but these devices are important in helping people walk independently and avoid falling. Many Parkinson's patients also benefit from physical therapy. Physical therapists can teach strengthening and stretching exercises that help Parkinson's patients stand up straighter and improve their walking. These exercises can also

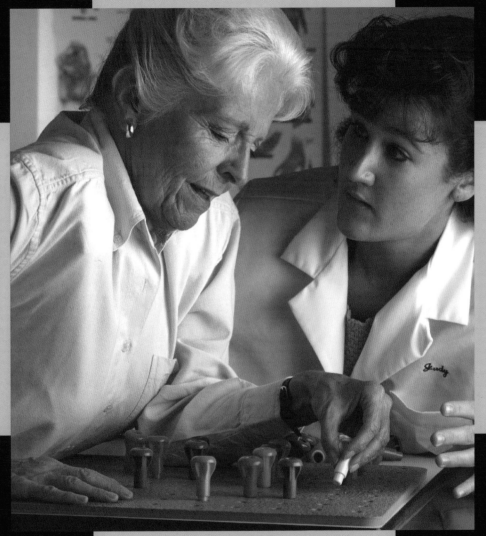

Physical therapists can help people regain the use of muscles stiffened by disease or condition.

Discovering Levodopa

After World War I (1914–18), an **epidemic** of encephalitis lethargica, otherwise known as sleeping sickness, swept the globe, infecting as many as 5 million people. As a result of the disease, most people developed a condition similar to Parkinson's. Many lost the ability to walk and talk and were institutionalized for decades, trapped in their own bodies. In 1966, neurologist Oliver Sacks began to treat some of these patients at Beth Abraham Hospital in New York with a new drug called levodopa. Almost overnight, the patients went from being in a comatose state, in which they appeared awake but were unconscious, to being able to play baseball. Although many of the patients who were treated with levodopa suffered setbacks and returned to their previous condition, the experience led to more refined research and the use of levodopa in Parkinson's patients. Today, the drug remains one of the most effective treatments for relieving the symptoms of Parkinson's disease.

help to keep pain under control, while breathing and relaxation techniques can reduce anxiety. Some clinics and health clubs have classes specifically for people with Parkinson's.

Therapy alone is often not enough to control the effects of Parkinson's. Several medications are available to treat the symptoms of the disease. Doctors disagree about the best time to begin treating Parkinson's, but in general, physicians will wait to prescribe medication until a person's symptoms interfere with daily functioning, since drug treatments can lose their effectiveness over time. Such a course is of particular concern to young-onset patients, who might live for several decades with the disease.

Because low levels of dopamine seem to lead to Parkinson's, it might seem logical to treat the disease by giving patients dopamine supplements. But, although the brain produces dopamine, a protective shield called the blood-brain barrier prevents dopamine in the blood from reaching the brain. To bypass this barrier, doctors often prescribe a combination of two drugs called levodopa and carbidopa. When a patient takes levodopa, the body converts the drug into dopamine in the bloodstream, rendering it unable to pass through the blood-brain barrier. Carbidopa, however, helps keep the levodopa from being converted into dopamine while in the blood, allowing the drug to enter the brain and boost levels of the neurotransmitter.

Other drugs have also been developed to treat Parkinson's. Amantadine, a drug originally designed to fight influenza, can reduce some of the involuntary movements typical of early Parkinson's. Monoamine oxidase inhibitors, which are powerful antidepressants, help the limited dopamine in Parkinson's patients' brains work longer and enhance the effect of levodopa. Other drugs called dopamine agonists mimic dopamine in the brain and are sometimes prescribed for patients early in the course of the disease to delay the start of levodopa treatment.

Drug therapies are not only expensive, costing Parkinson's patients roughly $2,500 a year, but they can also cause unwanted side effects. People taking drug therapy might suffer from nausea, trouble concentrating and remembering, **hallucinations**, sleep changes, and low blood pressure. They might also develop dyskinesia—involuntary movements, such as fidgeting or wiggling, that are different from the tremors caused by Parkinson's. Another problem is that the effectiveness of the drugs can change throughout the day. When the medication is doing its job, Parkinson's patients are said to be experiencing "on" times. If the medicine is not working, the patient is having an "off" time. This on-and-off behavior can make patients feel as if they have a switch in their heads that they cannot control.

Parkinson's disease levels a heavy financial impact on patients and taxpayers. The direct costs (such as treatment) combined with indirect costs (including the lost income from not being able to work) add up to an estimated $66 million per day in the U.S.

In the brain scan image opposite, the globus pallidus is the most circular portion seen in the center of the brain.

When drug therapy ceases to relieve Parkinson's symptoms, or if the side effects become too severe, some patients become candidates for brain surgery. In a pallidotomy, a surgeon inserts a hollow probe into the globus pallidus, a circular area deep inside the brain that helps to regulate voluntary movements. The probe destroys a portion of the globus pallidus and reduces overactive communication between nerve cells to help calm tremors, rigidity, and involuntary jerky movements. The surgery is not without risk, however; unsuccessful surgeries can cause vision damage, paralysis, or stroke.

Deep brain stimulation is a newer approach to the procedure. Instead of destroying brain tissue, the surgeon stimulates it by placing an **electrode** in the globus pallidus or an area nearby called the thalamus. The electrode is connected to a battery pack in the chest. Patients can turn the battery on and off by waving a special magnet over the location of the battery pack. When it's on, the device sends electrical impulses into the brain, blocking the overactive communication between nerve cells and calming symptoms such as tremor and rigidity. This procedure carries its own set of risks, including bleeding in the brain and infection.

Although medications and surgery can help treat the physical symptoms of Parkinson's, patients often suffer from mental and emo-

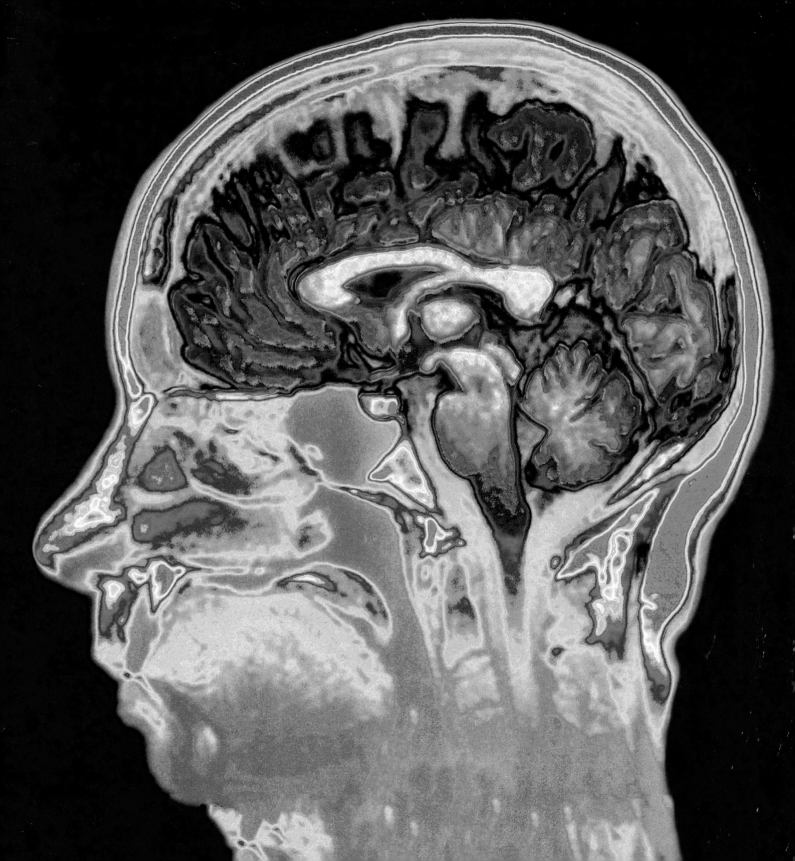

For some people with Parkinson's, the medication that relieves symptoms causes other problems. About 30 percent of patients report having visual hallucinations as a result of medication. Roughly 5 to 10 percent experience false, paranoid, and bizarre thoughts as a result of their drug treatment.

tional problems as well. Roughly 30 percent of Parkinson's patients develop dementia or other memory and concentration problems that interfere with daily living. To keep their memory in shape, people with Parkinson's are encouraged to study crossword puzzles and play word and trivia games. Making "to do" lists and setting timers for when they need to take medication can provide external reminders.

Many people with Parkinson's also suffer from depression. Faced with a future of uncertainty and the loss of the life they once knew, Parkinson's patients can become overwhelmed easily. In addition, many of the symptoms of Parkinson's disease can cause patients to feel as if they are prisoners held captive in their own bodies. Sometimes, when they try to take a step down the sidewalk, they discover that they can't; their feet are frozen. Their facial muscles will not let them smile or look happy. The masked face, combined with the soft, **monotonous** voice of people with Parkinson's, can make it seem as if they are depressed even when they aren't. Many Parkinson's patients find it helpful to tell others that they are truly happy and friendly, even if they appear to be serious or angry. Such problems can be embarrassing, however, and patients might decide to avoid going out in public, which often leads to loneliness. Attending a support group can help patients overcome that loneliness.

CHAPTER FOUR

COMMITTED TO A CURE

In recent years, awareness of

Parkinson's disease has soared as many famous people have announced that they have the disease. When actor Michael J. Fox revealed his struggle with Parkinson's disease in 1998, he committed himself to finding a cure. His open dedication to Parkinson's research has helped shed new light on the disease. As a result, more funding has been put toward Parkinson's research. Since 2000, the Michael J. Fox Foundation has funded nearly $170 million in research, supporting projects that have studied everything from new methods of delivering drugs to the brain to new clues, or biomarkers, within the body that might indicate that a person is at risk of developing Parkinson's. In addition to the money provided by private research foundations, in 2008, the National Institutes of Health funded $86 million in Parkinson's research, including studies to evaluate possible environmental and genetic causes of the disease and ways to improve diagnostic accuracy.

The Parkinson's Action Network (PAN) also works to raise awareness of Parkinson's disease and the issues people with the disease face.

Spearheaded by its namesake, the Michael J. Fox Foundation takes a targeted, multiple-step approach to researching a cure.

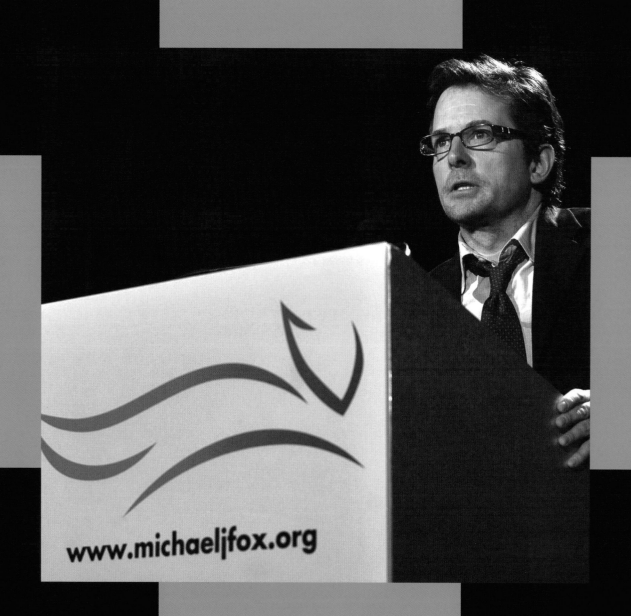

www.michaeljfox.org

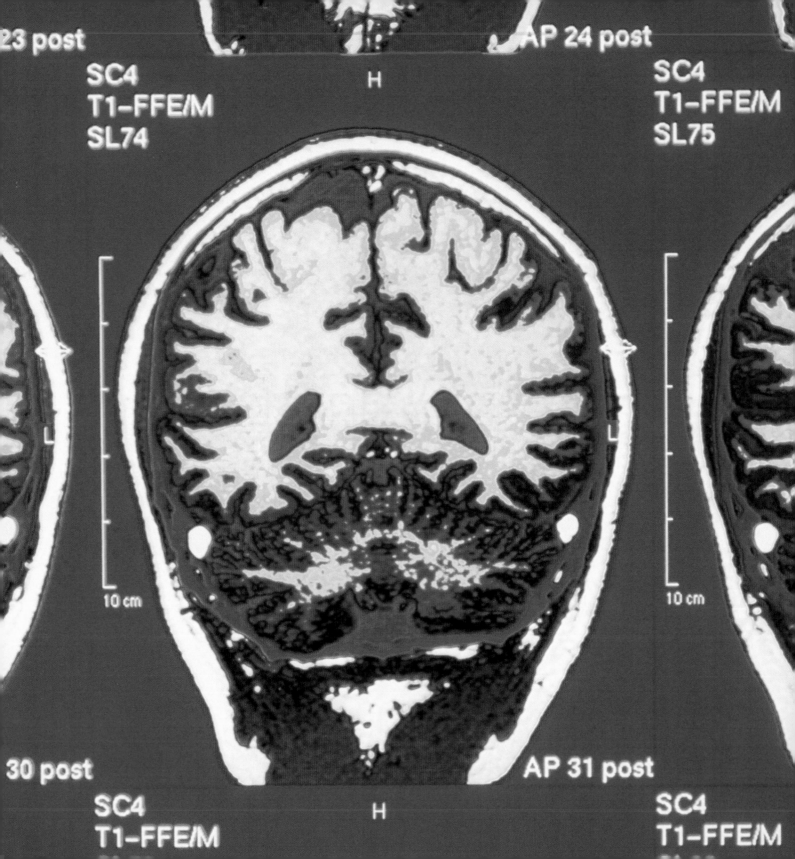

SC4
T1–FFE/M
SL74

H

SC4
T1–FFE/M
SL75

10 cm

10 cm

SC4
T1–FFE/M

H

SC4
T1–FFE/M

PARKINSON'S DISEASE

PAN supports the creation of a Parkinson's disease registry, a database of everyone in the U.S. with the condition. Currently, researchers do not know exactly how many people in the country have the disease. Having a registry that includes patients' names, geographic locations, ethnic backgrounds, ages, and family histories would help scientists identify trends in any of these groups. The data would also allow researchers to track changes over time.

Scientists continue to look for new ways to detect Parkinson's. New developments in X-ray and other imaging techniques have given physicians better tools for viewing the brain. Positron emission tomography (PET) scans, magnetic resonance imaging (MRI), and single-photon emission computerized tomography (SPECT) scans give views of the brain that are clearer than ever before. Researchers have studied a new type of MRI, known as diffusion tensor imaging (DTI), which has shown promise in distinguishing differences between the substantia nigra of people in the early stage of Parkinson's and those without the disease. The technology cannot yet identify the difference between Parkinson's and other disorders of the brain, but once researchers are able to see where the disease begins and how it affects the brain, they might be able to develop a cure or preventive measure. Imaging may also be a way to track the brain

A colored MRI scan can help doctors differentiate between the various parts of the brain.

as symptoms progress, which would allow doctors to know whether drug therapies are restoring the brain or protecting it from further damage.

One possibility for slowing the progression of Parkinson's could be the use of neuroprotective agents, which are substances that might shield the substantia nigra from damage. More than 10 possible neuroprotective agents, including caffeine, the **hormone** estrogen, and the dietary supplements coenzyme Q10 and creatine, are currently under research. Ibuprofen, sold over the counter to relieve headaches and other pains, is another possible neuroprotector. A study funded by the Michael J. Fox Foundation and the National Institute of Neurological Disorders and Stroke found in 2005 that people who took ibuprofen each day were 38 to 40 percent less likely to develop Parkinson's than those who did not take it.

Between 2001 and 2005, the pharmaceutical company Pfizer experimented with a voice-analysis computer program to pick up indications of the disease. The program compared earlier recordings of individuals with Parkinson's disease with recordings made after they had been diagnosed. It found that Parkinson's patients spoke in slight monotones many years before they developed other symptoms, although the voice change was too small to be detected by the human ear.

Men are roughly 50 percent more likely than women to develop Parkinson's disease. Scientists think this might be because men are more likely to come into contact with toxic substances and experience head trauma. Women also might receive protection against the disease from the hormone estrogen.

All in the Family

For many years, researchers believed that Parkinson's disease was caused largely by environmental factors, such as toxic chemicals, but over time, some began to suspect that people could inherit a tendency to develop the disease. In the 1980s, Dr. Roger Duvoisin of the Robert Wood Johnson Medical School in New Jersey studied a large Italian family of nearly 600 people who could all trace their ancestry to a single couple who had lived in Contursi, Italy, during the 18th century. Some of the descendants had immigrated to the U.S. between 1890 and 1920, while others remained in Italy. More than 60 members of the family in both countries had been diagnosed with Parkinson's disease. After studying the DNA of 28 family members, researchers were able to pinpoint the inherited gene **mutation** that they believed might have led to the development of Parkinson's disease. Those with the mutation had a 50 percent chance of passing it on to their children.

PARKINSON'S DISEASE

In addition to looking for new ways to diagnose Parkinson's, researchers are also enhancing the medications currently available to Parkinson's patients and developing new ways to treat symptoms. For example, the drug Parcopa, which was approved for use in the U.S. in 2004, is a combination of carbidopa and levodopa that dissolves in the mouth, which is helpful for those who have problems swallowing. In 2010, researchers at Beth Israel Deaconess Medical Center began a clinical trial using a therapy called repetitive transcranial magnetic stimulation (rTMS). The therapy involves placing a coil of plastic-coated wire over the scalp of a Parkinson's patient, which painlessly sends brief magnetic pulses through the skull and into the brain. These pulses temporarily change brain activity in the area to which they are delivered. For Parkinson's patients, researchers have studied using the procedure on the brain's motor cortex (at the top of the head) and the frontal lobe (behind the forehead). The study hoped to prove that rTMS could reduce the mood and motor symptoms in Parkinson's patients who had not been helped by medication and also suffered from depression.

Scientists have also studied stem cells for curing Parkinson's disease. While most cells cannot change (for example, a skin cell cannot be converted into a blood cell), stem cells can become any kind of cell anywhere in the body. Introducing stem cells into a sickly portion of the body could possibly stimulate a recovery as the healthy cells multiply and take over for sick ones. Theoretically, stem cells injected into the brains of people with Parkinson's could renew the dopamine-producing substantia nigra and bring about a recovery. Most stem cells used in research and treatments are adult stem cells (which are found in both children and adults). These cells usually come from **bone marrow** or the blood from an umbilical cord that connects a mother and baby until birth. However, the use of stem cells is **controversial** because some can come from extra **embryos** that have been scheduled to be discarded by fertility clinics. Harvesting embryonic stem cells has raised moral and ethical questions that researchers, patients, and the general public continue to debate.

Much has changed since the days when Parkinson's disease was known simply as the shaking palsy. The discovery of levodopa and other treatments has helped those suffering with the disease, but researchers continue to search for the missing pieces of the puzzle, including how to stop the disease's progression or reverse its effects. Ultimately, the goal of research is to find the cause. Once scientists can pinpoint the beginning of Parkinson's disease, they can work to end it.

Researchers estimate that the number of people worldwide with Parkinson's will swell to 8.7 million by the year 2030. They attribute this increase to improved identification of the disease, as well as a growing population of people aged 65 and older, who are more likely to develop it.

GLOSSARY

Alzheimer's disease: a condition, most often found in older people, in which brain matter and mental function are destroyed

autopsy: an examination of a body's vital organs after death to determine the cause of death

bone marrow: the tissue within bones where blood cells are created

chronic: lasting a long time or constantly recurring

comprehensive: large in scope; including many things

controversial: causing a dispute between two sides with opposing views

degenerative: causing a gradual decline in quality or deterioration of a part of the body

dementia: the deterioration of intellectual capability due to a disease of the brain

electrode: an object through which electricity enters or leaves something, such as a battery

embryos: human offspring in the early stages of development, from the time an egg is fertilized until the eighth week

epidemic: a disease that has spread rapidly through a segment of the population in a given geographic area

fetus: an unborn offspring of a mammal

genes: the basic units of instruction in a cell, which control a person's physical traits and pass characteristics from parents to offspring

hallucinations: perceptions of objects, sights, or sounds that do not exist

hormone: a substance produced by the body that affects activity within the body, such as growth

hypothesized: gave a possible explanation that could be tested by further investigation

involuntary: uncontrollable; not directed by the mind

monotonous: spoken in a single, unvaried tone of voice

mutation: a change in genetic material that is relatively permanent, resulting in a new characteristic or function in a cell

nervous system: a network in the body that includes the brain and the spinal cord; it determines responses to sensations and controls basic bodily functions such as the heartbeat

neurologist: a physician skilled in the diagnosis and treatment of diseases of the nervous system, including the brain

predisposition: a tendency or inclination to develop something, such as a disease

prognosis: a doctor's prediction regarding the probable course and outcome of a disease

protein: a complex structure that is the basic component of all living cells

spontaneously: happening all of a sudden without an apparent cause

stroke: a sudden attack caused by an interruption of blood supply to the brain that results in temporary or permanent disabilities

toxins: poisonous substances that can cause disease if they enter the body

unconscious: occurring without awareness

BIBLIOGRAPHY

Blake-Krebs, Barbara, and Linda Herman. *When Parkinson's Strikes Early: Voices, Choices, Resources, and Treatment.* Alameda, Calif.: Hunter House, 2001.

Bucher, Ric. "Grant Takes Charge of Parkinson's Battle." *ESPN.com,* May 18, 2009. http://sports.espn.go.com/espn/print?id=4174877&type=story.

Christensen, Jackie Hunt. *The First Year—Parkinson's Disease: An Essential Guide for the Newly Diagnosed.* New York: Marlowe & Company, 2005.

Fox, Michael J. *Lucky Man: A Memoir.* New York: Hyperion, 2002.

Friedman, Joseph H. *Making the Connection Between Brain and Behavior: Coping with Parkinson's Disease.* New York: Demos Health, 2008.

McGoon, Dwight. *The Parkinson's Handbook.* New York: W. W. Norton & Company, 1990.

National Parkinson Foundation. "Parkinson's Disease Overview." National Parkinson Foundation. http://www.parkinson.org/parkinson-s-disease.aspx.

Weiner, William, Lisa Shulman, and Anthony Lang. *Parkinson's Disease: A Complete Guide for Patients and Families.* Baltimore, Md.: Johns Hopkins University Press, 2001.

FURTHER READING

Goldstein, Natalie. *Parkinson's Disease.* New York: Chelsea House, 2009.

Landau, Elaine. *Parkinson's Disease.* New York: Franklin Watts, 1999.

Payment, Simone. *Michael J. Fox: Parkinson's Disease Research Advocate.* New York: Rosen Publishing Group, 2009.

Stoyles, Pennie. *The A–Z of Health.* Vol. 5, P–S. North Mankato, Minn.: Smart Apple Media, 2011.

INDEX

Ali, Muhammad 12
  Muhammad Ali Parkinson
    Center 12
Brain functioning 4, 8, 16, 18,
    19, 21, 29, 30, 32, 39,
    40, 44
  as affected by Parkinson's 4, 8,
    16, 18, 32
  nerve cells 16, 18, 19, 21, 32
  neurotransmitters 16, 18, 19,
    21, 29, 30, 44
    dopamine 16, 18, 19, 21,
      29, 30, 44
    norepinephrine 18
    serotonin 18
    proteins 18
      Lewy bodies 18
  substantia nigra 16, 18, 19,
    21, 39, 40, 44
  testing of 39
  and toxins 19, 21
brain surgery 32
Caretaking 25
causes 8, 12, 19, 20, 21, 41,
    42, 44
  environmental factors 19, 21,
    41, 42
  head trauma 12, 19, 41

possible genetic connection 19,
    20, 21, 42
Charot, Jean Martin 6
Death rates 24, 25
  and complications from
    Parkinson's 24, 25
degenerative nature 8, 26
diagnosis 4, 8, 10, 11, 14, 36,
    39, 40, 42, 43
  age at 4, 8
  and brain imaging 39
  four signs to determine 10, 11,
    14
  and gene mutations 42
  posthumous confirmation 10
drug treatments 6, 22, 25, 28,
    29–30, 31, 32, 34, 40,
    43, 44
  amantadine 30
  antidepressants 30
  carbidopa 29, 43
  cost 30, 31
  levodopa 6, 28, 29, 30, 43,
    44
  Parcopa 43
  side effects 30, 32, 34
Duvoisin, Roger 42
Fox, Michael J. 22, 36, 40

Michael J. Fox Foundation 36,
    40
Genes 19, 42
Grant, Brian 4
Hitler, Adolf 14
Life expectancies with Parkinson's
    25, 29
Nervous system disorders 10, 15
  Alzheimer's disease 15
  multiple sclerosis 10, 15
neurologists 4, 6, 21, 28
number of people affected 8, 15,
    20, 45
  future projections 45
Parkinson, James 6
parkinsonism 14, 28
Parkinson's Action Network 36, 39
  and creation of disease registry
    39
progression 10, 11, 21, 25, 26,
    40, 41, 44
  and neuroprotective agents 40,
    41
  scales for measuring 21, 25
    Hoehn and Yahr 21, 25
    Unified Parkinson's Disease
      Rating 21
  stages 21, 25

Research efforts 6, 18, 22, 36,
    39, 40, 43–44
  on causes 36, 44
  neurotransmitters 18
  rTMS clinical trials 43
  search for a cure 22, 36, 39,
    43–44
    and stem cells 43–44
  treatments 36, 40, 43
Sacks, Oliver 28
support groups 35
symptoms 4, 6, 8, 9, 10, 11, 12,
    14, 18, 21, 22, 25, 26, 28,
    29, 30, 32, 34, 35, 39, 43
  balance loss 10, 14, 25
  dementia 9, 18, 35
  depression 8, 9, 35, 43
  muscle rigidity 6, 8, 10, 11,
    14, 18, 22, 32
    cogwheel 11
    lead-pipe 11
  slow movements 10, 11, 12,
    14, 25
  tremors 4, 6, 8, 10, 12, 22,
    25, 30, 32
Therapy 25, 26, 29
Young-onset Parkinson's 4, 8, 10,
    22, 26, 29

Published by Creative Education • P.O. Box 227, Mankato, Minnesota 56002
Creative Education is an imprint of The Creative Company
www.thecreativecompany.us
Design and production by The Design Lab • Art direction by Rita Marshall
Printed by Corporate Graphics in the United States of America
Photographs by Alamy (Alan King Engraving, Peter Arnold, Inc.), Corbis (Peter Saloutos), Getty
Images (AFP, Barros & Barros, Andrew D. Bernstein/NBAE, Steve Gschmeissner/SPL, Kevin
Mazur/MJF/Wirelmage, The Science Picture Company, Moritz Steiger)

Library of Congress Cataloging-in-Publication Data
Dittmer, Lori. Parkinson's disease / by Lori Dittmer. p. cm. — (Living with disease)
Includes bibliographical references and index. Summary: A look at Parkinson's disease, examining
the ways in which it develops, its symptoms and diagnosis, the effects it has on a person's daily
life, and research toward finding better treatments.
ISBN 978-1-60818-076-9
1. Parkinson's disease—Juvenile literature. I. Title.
RC382.D58 2011   616.8'33—dc22   2010030366

CPSIA: 110310 PO1384
First Edition 9 8 7 6 5 4 3 2 1